CW00473873

The Sirtfood Diet Cookbook for Breakfast Lovers

50 Fast, Simple, and Tasty Recipes to Start the Day, Burn Fat and Boost your Metabolism

Anne Patel

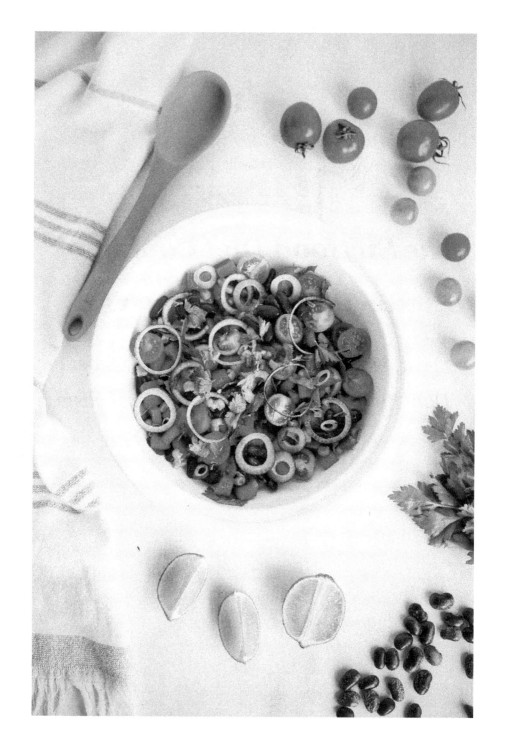

© Copyright 2021 - All rights reserved.

The content contained within this book may not be reproduced, duplicated or transmitted without direct written permission from the author or the publisher.

Under no circumstances will any blame or legal responsibility be held against the publisher, or author, for any damages, reparation, or monetary loss due to the information contained within this book. Either directly or indirectly.

Legal Notice:

This book is copyright protected. This book is only for personal use. You cannot amend, distribute, sell, use, quote or paraphrase any part, or the content within this book, without the consent of the author or publisher.

Disclaimer Notice:

Please note the information contained within this document is for educational and entertainment purposes only. All effort has been executed to present accurate, up to date, and reliable, complete information. No warranties of any kind are declared or implied. Readers acknowledge that the author is not engaging in the rendering of legal, financial, medical or professional advice. The content within this book has been derived from various sources. Please consult a licensed professional before attempting any techniques outlined in this book.

By reading this document, the reader agrees that under no circumstances is the author responsible for any losses, direct or indirect, which are incurred as a result of the use of information contained within this document, including, but not limited to, — errors, omissions, or inaccuracies.

Table of Contents

Chapter 1: What is the Sirtfood diet 8

Chapter 2: How do the Sirtfood Diet Works?........................19

50 Essential Breakfast Recipes 24

   1. Soy Berry Smoothie 24

   2. Paleolicious Smoothie Bowl 25

   3. Banana-Peanut Butter 'n Greens Smoothie.................... 28

   4. Fruity Tofu Smoothie 29

   5. Green Vegetable Smoothie 31

   6. Creamy Oats, Greens & Blueberry Smoothie.................... 32

   7. Potato Bites...33

   8. Sesame Dip..35

   9. Rosemary Squash Dip 36

   10. Bean Spread.. 38

   11. Carrots and Cauliflower Spread................................. 39

   12. Italian Veggie Salsa...41

   13. Sweet Oatmeal 43

   14. Green Beans and Eggs 45

   15. Spiced Morning Omelet... 48

   16. Rice Pudding... 50

   17. Creamy Millet...53

18. Apple Muffins...55

19. Mushroom Frittata..57

20. Homemade Granola Bowl 60

21. Steak with Veggies..62

22. Shrimp with Veggies 64

23. Chickpeas with Swiss Chard 66

24. Buckwheat Noodles with Chicken 68

25. Spicy Sesame & Edamame Noodles 70

26. Triple Berry Millet Bake 72

27. Green Shakshuka 74

28. Kale and Butternut Bowls.............................77

29. Egg Casserole 79

30. Vegan Tofu Omelet....................................... 81

31. Grapefruit & Celery Blast 84

32. Orange & Celery Crush 85

33. Tropical Chocolate Delight 87

34. Walnut & Spiced Apple Tonic........................88

35. Sweet Rocket (Arugula) Boost 89

36. Banana & Ginger Snap...................................90

37. Chocolate, Strawberry & Coconut Crush......... 91

38. Chocolate Berry Blend..................................92

39. Cranberry & Kale Crush 94

40. Poached Eggs & Rocket (Arugula) 95

41. Strawberry Buckwheat Pancakes 97

42. Strawberry & Nut Granola 98

43. Chilled Strawberry & Walnut Porridge 100

44. Fruit & Nut Yogurt Crunch 101

45. Cheesy Baked Eggs 102

46. Spiced Scramble 103

47. Sirtfood Mushroom Scramble Eggs 104

48. Blue Hawaii Smoothie 106

49. Turkey Breakfast Sausages 107

50. Banana Pecan Muffins 108

Chapter 1: What is the Sirtfood diet

The Sirtfood Diet was created by Masters in Nutritional Medicine, Aiden Goggins and Glen Matten.

Their goal initially was to find a healthier way for people to eat, but people started losing weight quickly when they tested their program. With all the people in the world following diets hoping to lose pounds, they thought it would be selfish not to disclose their innovative health plan.

The plan they developed focuses on combining certain foods eaten in order to maximize the supply of nutrition to our body. There is an initial phase in which calories are limited to give the body a period to recover and eliminate accumulated waste. A maintenance phase follows this first phase to accustom the metabolism to the new foods you are ingesting. Throughout all stages, you will incorporate potent green juices and well-structured, well-planned meals.

The diet focuses on so-called 'sirtfoods,' plant-based foods that are known to stimulate a gene called sirtuin in the human body.

Sirtuins belong to an entire protein family, called SIRT1 to SIRT7, and each has specific health-related connections. These proteins help separate and safeguard our cells from inflammation and other damage resulting from everyday activities, helping to reduce our risk of developing major diseases, particularly those related to aging.

Studies have shown that people live longer and healthier lives when they eat diets rich in these foods that activate sirtuin, free from diabetes, heart disease, and even dementia. So this diet was designed to restore a healthy body situation, and one of the byproducts of a healthy body is also the loss of excess weight.

The diet Sirtfood is neither a miracle cure nor a week-long program designed to quickly lose weight before beach holidays. If you are only interested in losing a few pounds and then returning to your old habits, there are certainly plans and diets that are more suited to your needs.

The Sirtfood diet is a project born to help you for the rest of your life, using delicious foods, but that will also improve your health. If you switch from a standard American diet (SAD) to a sirtfood diet, you will lose all the weight your body does not need.

A healthy body does not store extra energy. It asks for what it needs and uses it effectively.

The diet isn't designed to encourage you to starve or deprive yourself. The fact is, foods that are deficient in nutrients are designer made to deprive you and, though the calories are there in plenty, your cells are still starved for the nutrition to help you thrive. The Sirtfood Diet is the opposite of deprivation and starvation. It is nourishment and balance.

Most people following the SAD may use 20 ingredients in a month, let alone enjoy the sheer volume of choice ingredients from the 120 options you will learn about here.

In recent decades, an alarming number of people have come to the conclusion that healthy food is boring, and plants or, more specifically, vegetables are terrible tasting. This is because the foods we've become dependent on – packed with sugar, salt, and unhealthy fats – have chemically altered our connection to food. Our brains are essentially lying to us, and our taste buds have been compromised.

This is one of the reasons the week-long reset is so important. After this first week, you will be able to taste food differently. The more you expose yourself to the recommended plant-based foods, the more pleasure you get out of them.

Sirtuins are critical for our health, regulating many essential biological functions, including our metabolism, which, I'm sure you know, is very closely connected to our weight. It's also a key figure in determining our body composition, such as how much muscle we build and how much fat we retain.

Sirtuin genes regulate all this and more. They're also integral in the process of aging and disease.

If we can turn these genes on, we'll be able to protect our cells and enjoy better health for longer life. Eating sirtfoods is the most effective way to accomplish this goal.

Sirtfoods are all plant-based, and they have many more benefits, in addition to being sirtuin activators.

Our bodies require energy to operate, and the majority of this fuel comes from three primary macronutrients: carbohydrates, fats, and proteins. These macros largely control our metabolic system and regulate how the calories we consume get processed by our bodies. This is why most diets focus exclusively on micronutrition and require you to calculate calories.

Our bodies need more than just energy to survive than thriving, however, which is why micronutrients are so important. They don't impact our weight as obviously as macros, but they are our health foundations.

Micronutrients, such as vitamins, minerals, fiber, antioxidants, and phytonutrients, are supposed to be consumed along with our calories. Unfortunately, in the Standard American Diet (SAD), they're in very limited supply.

When your diet is primarily made up of large quantities of red meat and processed meats, pre-packaged foods, vegetable oils, refined grains and a lot of sugar, you will have an almost total lack of micronutrition.

Plant foods offer the most micronutrients per calorie consumed. Every edible plant has a unique nutritional profile, protecting you from an innumerable variety of illnesses.

Sirtfoods, and other plant-based sources of nutrition, give your body what it needs to stay young and disease-free, and, as a bonus, this will help you remain at an ideal weight.

The original Sirtfood Diet encourages you to commit to a one week reset phase and then a 2-week maintenance phase where you rely heavily on the Sirtfood green juice for a significant dose of nutrition along with meals rich in sirtfoods. Once the phases are complete, to retain your health for the rest of your life, you will need to continue incorporating these sirtfoods into your daily meals.

The Sirtfood Diet is not a miracle cure, but if you stick to these recipes, you'll not just impress your taste buds, but you'll also enhance nearly every aspect of your health. To get safe, you don't have to count calories or starve yourself, the youthful body you've always wanted.

Sirtfood Diet Phases

Every newbie needs to understand that the sirtfood diet does not start with a single list of ingredients in your hands. Its implementation and adaptation are more than mere selective grocery shopping. Every diet can only work effectively when we allow our body to embrace the sudden shift and change in food intake. Similarly, the sirtfood diet also comes with two phases of adaptation. If a dieter successfully goes through these phases, he can continue with the sirtfood diet easily. There are mainly two phases of this diet, which are then succeeded by a third phase in which you can decide how you want to continue the diet.

<u>Phase One</u>

The first seven days of this diet plan are characterized as Phase One. In this phase, a dieter must focus on calorie restriction and the intake of green juices. These seven days are crucial to initiate your weight loss and usually help to lose up to seven pounds if the diet is followed properly. If you find yourself achieving this target, that means that you are on the right track.

In the first three days of the first phase, a dieter must restrict this caloric intake to 1,000 calories only. While doing so, the dieter must also have green juice throughout the day, probably three times a day. Try to drink green juice per meal. The recipes given in the book are perfect for selecting from.

Many meal options can keep your caloric intake in checks, such as buckwheat noodles, seared tofu, some shrimp stir fry, or sirtfood omelet.

Once the first three days of this diet has passed, you can increase your caloric intake to 1,500 calories per day. In these next four days, you can reduce the green juices to two times per side. And pair the juices with more Sirtuin-rich food in every meal.

Phase Two

After the first week of the sirtfood diet, then starts phase two. This phase is more about the maintenance of the diet, as the first week enables the body to embrace the change and start working according to the new diet. This phase enables the body to continue working towards the weight loss objective slowly and steadily. Therefore, the duration of this phase is almost two weeks.

So how is this phase different from phase one? In this phase, there is no restriction on the caloric intake, as long as the food is rich in sirtuins and you are taking it three times a day, it is good to go. Instead of having the green juice two or three times a day, the dieter can have juice one time a day, and that will be enough to achieve steady weight loss. You can have the juice after any meal, in the morning or in the evening.

After the Diet Phase

With the end of phase two comes the time, which is most crucial, and that is the after-diet phase. If your weight loss target has not been reached by the end of step two, then you can restart the phases all over again. Or even when you have achieved the goals but still want to lose more weight, then you can again give it a try.

Instead of following phases one and two over and over again, you can also continue having good quality sirtfood meals in this after-diet phase. Simply continue the eating practices of phase two, have a diet rich in sirtuin and do have green juices whenever possible. The diet is mainly divided into two phases: the first lasts one week, and the other lasts 14 days.

The best 20 sirt foods

All these foods include high quantities of plant compounds called polyphenols, which can be thought to modify the sirtuin enzymes, therefore, excite their super-healthy added benefits.

Top 20 sirtfoods

1. Arugula (Rocket)
2. Buckwheat
3. Capers
4. Celery
5. Chilis
6. Cocoa
7. Coffee
8. Extra Virgin Olive Oil
9. Garlic
10. Green Tea (especially Matcha)
11. Kale
12. Medjool Dates
13. Parsley
14. Red Endive
15. Red Onions
16. Red Wine
17. Soy
18. Strawberries

19. Turmeric

20. Walnuts

What Is So Great About Sirtuins?

There are seven types of Sirtuins named from **SIRT1** to **SIRT7**. Although our understanding of the exact functions of all the Sirtuins is minimal, studies show that activating them can have the following benefits:

Switching on fat burning and protection from weight gain: Sirtuins do this by increasing the mitochondrion's functionality (which is involved in the production of energy) and sparking a change in your metabolism to break down more fat cells.

Improving Memory by protecting neurons from damage. Sirtuins also boost learning skills and memory through the enhancement of synaptic plasticity. Synaptic plasticity refers to synapses' capacity to weaken or strengthen with time due to decreased or increased activity. This is important because memories are represented by different interconnected networks of synapses in the brain, and synaptic plasticity is an important neurochemical foundation of memory and learning.

Slowing down the Ageing Process: Sirtuins act as cell guarding enzymes. Thus, they protect the cells and slow down their aging process.

Repairing cells: The Sirtuins repair cells damaged by re-activating cell functionality.

Protection against diabetes: this happens through prevention against insulin resistance. Sirtuins do this by controlling blood sugar levels because this diet calls for moderate consumption of carbohydrates. These foods cause increases in blood sugar levels; hence the need to release insulin, and as the blood sugar levels increase greatly, there is a need to produce more insulin. Over time, cells become resistant to insulin, hence producing more insulin and leading to insulin resistance.

Fighting Cancers: The chemicals working as sirtuin activators affect the function of sirtuin in different cells, i.e. by switching it on when in normal cells and shutting it down in cancerous cells. This encourages the death of cancerous cells.

Fighting inflammation: Sirtuins have a powerful antioxidant effect that has the power to reduce oxidative stress. This has positive effects on heart health and cardiovascular protection.

Chapter 2: How do the Sirtfood Diet Works?

The basis of the sirtuin diet can be explained in simple terms or in complex ways. However, it's important to understand how and why it works so that you can appreciate the value of what you are doing. It is important to also know why these sirtuin rich foods help to help you maintain fidelity to your diet plan. Otherwise, you may throw something in your meal with less nutrition that would defeat the purpose of planning for one rich in sirtuins. Most importantly, this is not a dietary fad, and as you will see, there is much wisdom contained in how humans have used natural foods, even for medicinal purposes, over thousands of years.

To understand how the Sirtfood diet works and why these particular foods are necessary, we're going to look at their role in the human body.

Sirtuin activity was first researched in yeast, where a mutation caused an extension in the yeast's lifespan. Sirtuins were also shown to slow aging in laboratory mice, fruit flies, and nematodes. As research on Sirtuins proved to transfer to mammals, they were examined for their use in diet and slowing the aging process. The sirtuins in humans are different in typing, but they essentially work in the same ways and reasons.

The Sirtuin family is made up of seven "members." It is believed that sirtuins play a big role in regulating certain functions of cells, including proliferation, reproduction and growth of cells), apoptosis death of cells). They promote survival and resist stress to increase longevity.

They are also seen to block neurodegeneration loss or function of the nerve cells in the brain). They conduct their housekeeping functions by cleaning out toxic proteins and supporting the brain's ability to change and adapt to different conditions or to recuperate i.e., brain plasticity). They also help minimize chronic inflammation as part of this and decrease anything called oxidative stress. Oxidative stress is when there are so many free radicals present in the body that are cell-damaging, and by fighting them with antioxidants, the body can not keep up. These factors are related to age-related illness and weight as well, which again brings us back to a discussion of how they actually work.

You will see labels in Sirtuins that start with "SIR," which represents "Silence Information Regulator" genes. They do exactly that, silence or regulate, as part of their functions. Humans work with the seven sirtuins: SIRT1, SIRT2, SIRT3,

SIRT4, SIRT 5, SIRT6 and SIRT7. Each of these types is responsible for different areas of protecting cells. They work by either stimulating or turning on certain gene expressions or by reducing and turning off other gene expressions. This essentially means that they can influence genes to do more or less of something, most of which they are already programmed to do.

Through enzyme reactions, each of the SIRT types affects different areas of cells responsible for the metabolic processes that help maintain life. This is also related to what organs and functions they will affect.

For example, the SIRT6 causes and expression of genes in humans that affect skeletal muscle, fat tissue, brain, and heart. SIRT 3 would cause an expression of genes that affect the kidneys, liver, brain and heart.

If we tie these concepts together, you can see that the Sirtuin proteins can change the expression of genes, and in the case of the Sirtfood diet, we care about how sirtuins can turn off those genes that are responsible for speeding up aging and for weight management.

The other aspect to this conversation of sirtuins is the function and the power of calorie restriction on the human body. Calorie restriction is simply eating fewer calories. This, coupled with exercise and reducing stress, is usually a combination for weight loss. Calorie restriction has also proven across much research in animals and humans to increase one's lifespan.

We can look further at the role of sirtuins with calorie restriction and using the SIRT3 protein, which has a role in metabolism and aging. Amongst all of the effects of the protein on gene expression, such as preventing cells from dying, reducing tumors from growing, etc.), we want to understand the effects of SIRT3 on weight for this book's purpose.

As we stated earlier, the SIRT3 has high expression in those metabolically active tissues, and its ability to express itself increases with caloric restriction, fasting, and exercise. On the contrary, it will express itself less when the body has high fat, high calorie-riddled diet.

The last few highlights of sirtuins are their role in regulating telomeres and reducing inflammation, which also helps with staving off disease and aging.
Telomeres are sequences of proteins at the ends of chromosomes. When cells divide, these get shorter. As we age, they get shorter, and other stressors to the body also will contribute to this. Maintaining these longer telomeres is the key to slower aging. In addition, proper diet, along with exercise and other variables, can lengthen telomeres. SIRT6 is one of the

sirtuins that, if activated, can help with DNA damage, inflammation and oxidative stress. SIRT1 also helps with inflammatory response cycles that are related to many age-related diseases.

Calories restriction can extend life to some degree. Since this and fasting are a stressor, these factors will stimulate the SIRT3 proteins to kick in and protect the body from the stressors and excess free radicals. Again, the telomere length is affected as well.

Having laid this all out before you, you should appreciate how and why these miraculous compounds work in your favor, keep you youthful, healthy, and lean If they are working hard for you, don't you feel that you should do something too?

50 Essential Breakfast Recipes

1. Soy Berry Smoothie

Preparation time: 5 minutes.
Cooking time: 0 minutes.
Serving: 1

Ingredients:
1 cup fresh strawberries/blueberries or frozen
1 cup unsweetened vanilla soymilk

Directions:
Blend or blitz all the ingredients. Enjoy.

Nutrition:
Calories: 260cal
Carbs: 44g
Sugar: 34g
Fat: 4.5g

2. Paleolicious Smoothie Bowl

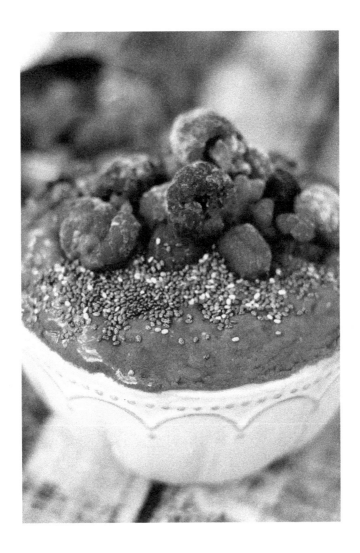

Preparation time: 5 minutes.

Cooking time: 0 minutes.

Serving: 1

Ingredients:

1 piece banana (frozen)

1 hand spinach

1/2 pieces mango

1/2 pieces avocado

100 milliliters almond milk

For garnish:

½ pieces mango

1 hand raspberries

1 tablespoon grated coconut

1 tablespoon walnuts, roughly chopped

Directions:

1. In a blender, place the ingredients and combine to an even mass

2. Put the mixture in a bowl and garnish with the remaining ingredients.

3. Of course, you can vary the garnish as you wish.

Nutrition:

Calories: 180cal

Carbs: 42g

Sugar: 30g

Fat: 31.5g

3. Banana-Peanut Butter 'n Greens Smoothie

Preparation time: 5 minutes.
Cooking time: 0 minutes.
Servings: 1

Ingredients:
1 cup chopped and packed Romaine lettuce
1 frozen medium banana
1 tablespoon all-natural peanut butter
1 cup cold almond milk

Directions:
1. In a heavy-duty blender, add all the ingredients.

2. Puree until smooth and creamy.

3. Serve and enjoy.

Nutrition:
Calories: 349.3cal
Fat: 9.7g
Carbs: 57.4g
Protein: 8.1g

4. Fruity Tofu Smoothie

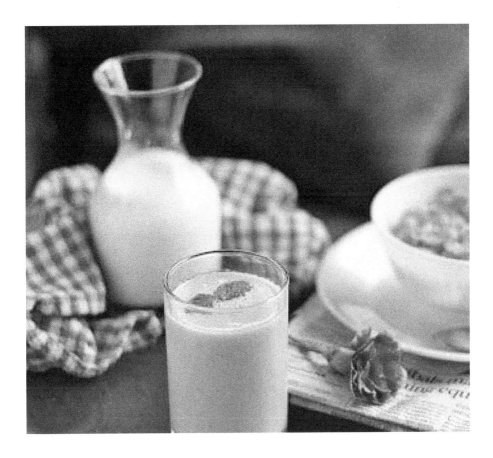

Preparation time: 5 minutes.

Cooking time: 0 minutes.

Servings: 2

Ingredients:

1 cup ice-cold water

1 cup packed spinach

¼ cup frozen mango chunks

½ cup frozen pineapple chunks

1 tablespoon chia seeds

1 container silken tofu

1 frozen medium banana

Directions:

1. Add all of the ingredients into a blender until smooth and fluffy.

2. Evenly divide into two glasses, serve, and enjoy.

Nutrition:

Calories: 175cal

Fat: 3.7g

Carbs: 33.3g

Protein: 6.0g

5. Green Vegetable Smoothie

Preparation time: 5 minutes.

Cooking time: 0 minutes.

Servings: 4

Ingredients:

1 cup cold water

½ cup strawberries

2 ounces baby spinach

1 lemon juice

1 tablespoon fresh mint

1 banana

½ cup blueberries

Directions:

1. Put the ingredients in a blender.

Nutrition:

Calories: 52cal

Fat: 2g

Carbs: 12g

Protein: 1g

6. Creamy Oats, Greens & Blueberry Smoothie

Preparation time: 4 minutes.

Cooking time: 0 minutes.

Servings: 1

Ingredients:

1 cup cold fat-free milk

1 cup salad greens

½ cup fresh frozen blueberries

½ cup frozen cooked oatmeal

1 tablespoon sunflower seeds

Directions:

1. In a blender, put all the ingredients until smooth and creamy.

2. Serve and enjoy.

Nutrition:

Calories: 280cal

Fat: 6.8g

Carbs: 44.0g

Protein: 14.0g

7. Potato Bites

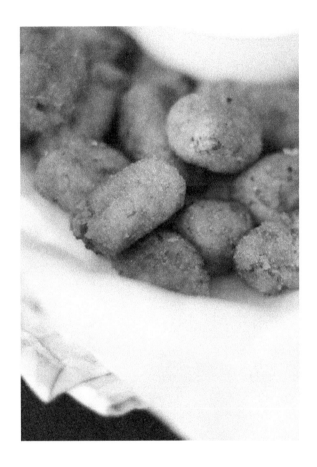

Preparation time: 10 minutes.

Cooking time: 20 minutes.

Servings: 4

Ingredients:

1 potato, sliced

2 bacon slices, already cooked and crumbled

1 small avocado, pitted and cubed

Cooking spray

Directions:

1. Spread potato slices on a lined baking sheet, spray with cooking oil, introduce in the oven at 350°F, bake for 20 minutes, arrange on a platter, top each slice with avocado and crumbled bacon and serve as a snack.

Nutrition:

Calories: 180cal

Fat: 4g

Fiber: 1g

Carbs: 8g

Protein: 6g

8. Sesame Dip

Preparation time: 10 minutes.
Cooking time: 0 minutes.
Servings: 4

Ingredients:

1 cup sesame seed paste, pure

Black pepper to taste

1 cup veggie stock

½ cup lemon juice

½ teaspoon cumin, ground

3 garlic cloves, chopped

Directions:

1. In your food processor, mix the sesame paste with black pepper, stock, lemon juice, cumin and garlic, pulse very well, divide into bowls and serve as a party dip.

Nutrition:

Calories: 120cal
Fat: 12g
Fiber: 2g
Carbs: 7g
Protein: 4g

9. Rosemary Squash Dip

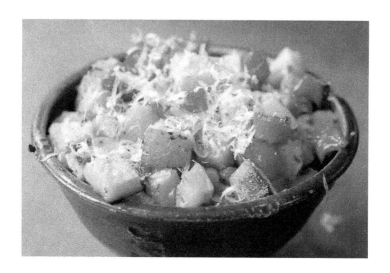

Preparation time: 10 minutes.

Cooking time: 40 minutes.

Servings: 4

Ingredients:

1 cup butternut squash, peeled and cubed

1 tablespoon water

Cooking spray

2 tablespoons coconut milk

2 teaspoons rosemary, dried

Black pepper to taste

Directions:

1. Spread squash cubes on a lined baking sheet, spray some cooking oil, introduce in the oven, bake at 365°F for 40 minutes, transfer to your blender, add water, milk, rosemary and black pepper, pulse well, divide into small bowls and serve.

Nutrition:
Calories: 182cal
Fat: 5g
Fiber: 7g
Carbs: 12g
Protein: 5g

10. Bean Spread

Preparation time: 10 minutes.

Cooking time: 7 hours.

Servings: 4

Ingredients:

1 cup white beans, dried

1 teaspoon apple cider vinegar

1 cup veggie stock

1 tablespoon water

Directions:

1. In your slow cooker, mix beans with stock, stir, cover, cook over low heat for 6 hours, drain, transfer to your food processor, add vinegar and water, pulse well, divide into bowls and serve.

Nutrition:

Calories: 181cal

Fat: 6g

Fiber: 5g

Carbs: 9g

Protein: 7g

11. Carrots and Cauliflower Spread

Preparation time: 10 minutes.
Cooking time: 40 minutes.
Servings: 4

Ingredients:
1 cup carrots, sliced
2 cups cauliflower florets
½ cup cashews
2 (½) cups water
1 cup almond milk
1 teaspoon garlic powder
¼ teaspoon smoked paprika

Directions:
1. In a small pot, mix the carrots with cauliflower, cashews and water, stir, cover, bring to a boil over medium heat, cook for 40 minutes, drain and transfer to a blender.

2. Add almond milk, garlic powder and paprika, pulse well, divide into small bowls and serve.

Nutrition:
Calories: 201cal

Fat: 7g
Fiber: 4g
Carbs: 7g
Protein: 7g

12. Italian Veggie Salsa

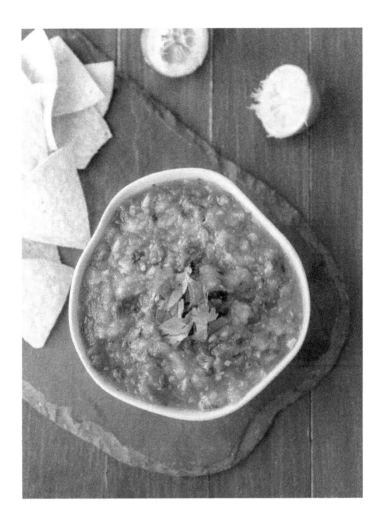

Preparation time: 10 minutes.

Cooking time: 10 minutes.

Servings: 4

Ingredients:

2 red bell peppers, cut into medium wedges

3 zucchinis, sliced

½ cup garlic, minced

2 tablespoons olive oil

A pinch of black pepper

1 teaspoon Italian seasoning

Directions:

1. Heat a pan with the oil over medium-high heat, add bell peppers and zucchini, toss and cook for 5 minutes.

2. Add garlic, black pepper and Italian seasoning, toss, cook for 5 minutes more, divide into small cups and serve as a snack.

Nutrition:

Calories: 132cal

Fat: 3g

Fiber: 3g

Carbs: 7g

Protein:4g

13. Sweet Oatmeal

Preparation Time: 5 minutes
Cooking Time: 10 minutes
Servings: 3

Ingredients:

1 cup oatmeal

5 apricots

1 tablespoon honey

1 cup coconut milk, unsweetened

1 teaspoon cashew butter

¼ teaspoon salt

½ cup of water

Directions:

1. Combine the coconut milk and oatmeal together in the saucepan and stir the mixture.

2. Add the water and stir it again. Sprinkle the mixture with the salt and close the lid.

3. Cook the oatmeal on medium heat for 10 minutes.

4. Meanwhile, chop the apricots into tiny pieces and combine the chopped fruit with the honey.

5. When the oatmeal is cooked, add cashew butter and fruit mixture.

6. Stir carefully and transfer to serving bowls.

7. Serve immediately.

Nutrition: Calories: 336, Fat: 21.2g, Total Carbs: 35.1g, Sugars: 14.0g,
Protein: 6.2g

14. Green Beans and Eggs

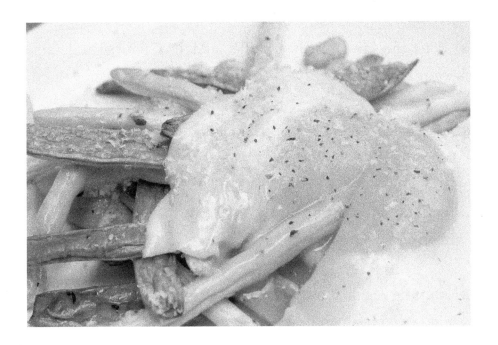

Preparation Time: 10 minutes

Cooking Time: 15 minutes

Servings: 2

Ingredients:

½ cup green beans

¼ teaspoon salt

5 eggs

1/3 cup skim milk

1 bell pepper, seeds removed

1 teaspoon olive oil

Directions:

1. Slice the bell pepper and combine it with the green beans.

2. Pour the olive oil in a skillet and transfer the vegetable mixture to the skillet.

3. Cook for 3 minutes over medium heat, stirring frequently. Meanwhile, beat the eggs in a mixing bowl.

4. Sprinkle the egg mixture with the salt and add skim milk. Whisk well.

5. Pour the egg mixture over the vegetable mixture and cook for 3 minutes on medium heat.

6. Stir the mixture carefully so that the eggs and vegetables are well combined.

7. Cook for 4 minutes more.

8. Stir again and close the lid.

9. Cook the scrambled eggs for 5 minutes more.

10. Stir the mixture again.

11. Serve it.

Nutrition: Calories: 231, Fat: 13.4g, Total Carbs: 9.3g, Sugars: 6.2g, Protein:16.3g

15. Spiced Morning Omelet

Preparation Time: 10 minutes
Cooking Time: 15 minutes
Servings: 3

Ingredients:

7 eggs

1/3 cup skim milk

3 garlic cloves

¼ teaspoon nutmeg

¼ teaspoon ground ginger

1 teaspoon cilantro

1 teaspoon olive oil

1 tablespoon chives

1 teaspoon turmeric

Directions:

1. Beat the eggs in a mixing bowl.

2. Add the skim milk and whisk again.

3. Sprinkle the egg mixture with the nutmeg, ground ginger, cilantro, and turmeric.

4. Peel the garlic cloves and mince them.

5. Chop the chives and combine with the minced garlic.

6. Add the herb mixture to the eggs and stir it again.

7. Preheat a skillet well and pour in the olive oil.

8. Preheat the olive oil over medium heat and then pour the egg mixture into the pan.

9. Close the lid and cook the omelet for 15 minutes.

10. When the dish is cooked, cool slightly and cut into the serving portions.

11. Serve it.

Nutrition: Calories: 179, Fat: 12.0g, Total Carbs: 3.8g, Sugars: 2.2g, Protein:14.1g

16. Rice Pudding

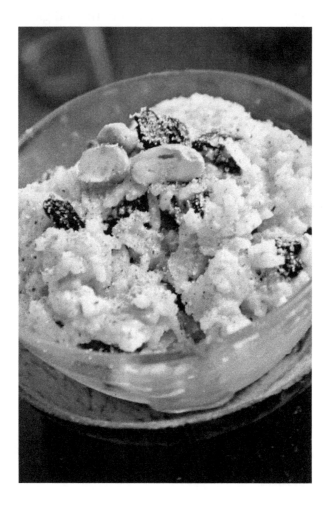

Preparation Time: 5 minutes

Cooking Time: 15 minutes

Servings: 5

Ingredients:

1 cup of brown rice

2 cups coconut milk, unsweetened

1 teaspoon cinnamon

1 teaspoon ginger

1/3 teaspoon thyme

1/3 cup almonds

2 tablespoon honey

1 teaspoon lemon zest

Directions:

1. Pour the coconut milk into a saucepan and heat until low.

2. Add the brown rice and stir the mixture carefully.

3. Close the lid and cook the brown rice over medium heat for 10 minutes.

4. Meanwhile, crush the almonds and combine them with the lemon zest, thyme, ginger, and cinnamon.

5. Sprinkle the brown rice with the almond mixture and stir it carefully.

6. Close the lid and cook the dish for 5 minutes.

7. Remove it from the saucepan when the pudding is cooked, and transfer it to a large bowl.

8. Add the honey and stir the pudding.

9. Serve it immediately.

Nutrition: Calories: 423, Fat: 27.1g, Total Carbs: 43.3g, Sugars: 10.4g, Protein: 6.5g

17. Creamy Millet

Preparation Time: 10 minutes
Cooking Time: 15 minutes
Servings: 8

Ingredients:

2 cups millet

1 cup almond milk, unsweetened

1 cup of water

1 cup coconut milk, unsweetened

1 teaspoon cinnamon

½ teaspoon ground ginger

¼ teaspoon salt

1 tablespoon chia seeds

1 tablespoon cashew butter

4 oz. Parmesan cheese, grated

Directions:

1. Combine the coconut milk, almond milk, and water together in the saucepan.

2. Stir the liquid gently and add millet.

3. Mix carefully and close the lid.

4. Cook the millet on the medium heat for 5 minutes.

5. Sprinkle the porridge with the cinnamon, ground ginger, salt, and chia seeds.

6. Carefully stir the mixture with a spoon and proceed to cook for 5 minutes more on medium heat.

7. Add the cashew butter and cook the millet for 5 minutes.

8. Remove the millet from the heat and transfer it to serving bowls.

9. Sprinkle the dish with the grated cheese.

10. Serve it.

Nutrition: Calories: 384, Fat: 19.8g, Total Carbs: 42.9g, Sugars: 3.6g, Protein: 11.7g

18. Apple Muffins

Preparation Time: 10 minutes
Cooking Time: 15 minutes
Servings: 5

Ingredients:

2 eggs

1 cup oat flour

½ teaspoon salt

2 tablespoon stevia

3 apples, washed and peeled

½ cup skim milk

1 tablespoon olive oil

½ teaspoon baking soda

1 teaspoon apple cider vinegar

Directions:

1. In the mixing bowl, beat and whisk the eggs well.

2. Add the skim milk, salt, baking soda, stevia, and apple cider vinegar.

3. Stir the mixture carefully.

4. Grate the apples and add the grated mixture in the egg mixture.

5. Stir it carefully and add the oat flour.

6. Add the olive oil and blend into a smooth batter

7. Preheat the oven to 350 F.

8. Fill each muffin from halfway with the batter and place the muffins in the oven.

9. Cook the dish for 15 minutes.

10. Remove the cooked muffins from the oven.

11. Cool the cooked muffins well and serve them.

Nutrition: Calories: 20, Fat: 6.0g, Total Carbs: 32.4g, Sugars: 15.3g, Protein:11.7g

19. Mushroom Frittata

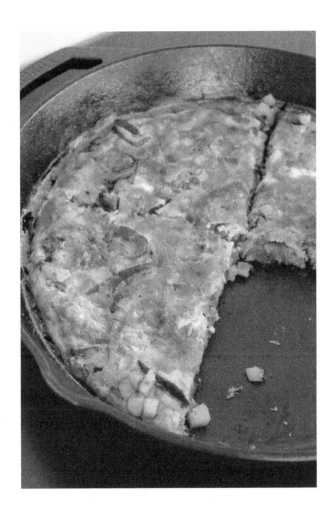

Preparation Time: 10 minutes

Cooking Time: 20 minutes

Servings: 5

Ingredients:

8 oz. shiitake mushrooms

1 teaspoon salt

1 cup broccoli

7 eggs

5 oz. Parmesan cheese

1 tablespoon olive oil

½ teaspoon ground ginger

5 garlic cloves

1 teaspoon oregano

1 teaspoon basil

1 teaspoon cilantro

½cuplow-

Fat milk

Directions:

1. Wash the shiitake mushrooms well and chop them.

2. Chop the broccoli and combine it with the mushrooms in a mixing bowl.

3. In a separate bowl, beat the eggs.

4. Sprinkle the egg mixture with the cilantro, basil, oregano, and ground ginger. Stir it well.

5. Add the low-Fat milk and broccoli. Stir the egg mixture well.

6. Peel the garlic cloves and mince them.

7. Add minced garlic in the egg mixture and stir it gently.

8. Preheat the oven to 350 F.

9. Spray a deep pan with olive oil

10. Into the pan, pour the egg mixture and put it in the preheated oven.

11. Cook the frittata for 20 minutes.

12. Remove it from the oven when the dish is baked, and cool slightly.

13. Serve the frittata immediately.

Nutrition: Calories: 250, Fat: 15.5g, Total Carbs: 11.5g, Sugars: 3.7g, Protein: 19.2g

20. Homemade Granola Bowl

Preparation Time: 10 minutes
Cooking Time: 20 minutes
Servings: 6

Ingredients:

3 tablespoons pumpkin seeds

1 tablespoon coconut oil

1 teaspoon sunflower seeds

¼ cup almonds

1 cup raw oats

3 tablespoons sesame seeds

5 tablespoons honey

2 cups almond milk, unsweetened

Directions:

1. Combine the pumpkin seeds, sunflower seeds, almonds, and sesame seeds together.

2. Crush the mixture well and add raw oats.

3. Add the honey and coconut oil.

4. Stir the mixture carefully until you get a smooth mix.

5. Preheat the oven to 350 F.

6. Cover the tray with parchment and transfer the seed mixture onto the tray. Flatten it well.

7. In the preheated oven, bring the tray in and cook for 20 minutes.

8. When the mixture is cooked, remove it from the oven and chill well.

9. Separate the mixture into small pieces and put in serving bowls.

10. Add the almond milk and mix up the dish.

11. Serve it.

Nutrition: Calories: 381, Fat: 28.5g, Total Carbs: 30.8g, Sugars: 17.4g, Protein: 6.4g

21. Steak with Veggies

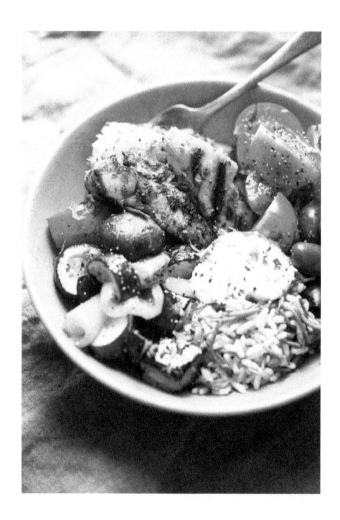

Preparation Time: 15 minutes

Cooking Time: 12 minutes

Servings: 4

Ingredients:

2 tablespoons coconut oil

4 garlic cloves, minced

1-pound beef sirloin steak, cut into bite-sized pieces Ground black pepper, as required

1½ cups carrots, peeled and cut into matchsticks 1½ cups fresh kale, tough ribs removed and chopped 3 tablespoons tamari

Directions:

1. Melt the coconut oil in a wok and sauté the garlic over medium heat for approximately 1 minute.

2. Add the beef and black pepper and stir to combine.

3. Increase the heat to medium-high and cook for about 3-4 minutes or until browned from all sides.

4. Add the carrot, kale and tamari and cook for about 4-5 minutes.

5. Remove from the heat and serve hot.

Nutrition: Calories 311 Total Fat 13.8 g Saturated Fat 8.6 g Cholesterol 101 mg Sodium 700 mg Total Carbs 8.4 g Fiber 1.6 g Sugar 2.3 g Protein 37.1 g

22. Shrimp with Veggies

Preparation Time: 15 minutes
Cooking Time: 8 minutes
Servings: 5

Ingredients:

For Sauce:

1 tablespoon fresh ginger, grated

2 garlic cloves, minced

3 tablespoons low-sodium soy sauce

1 tablespoon red wine vinegar

1 teaspoon brown sugar

¼ teaspoon red pepper flakes, crushed

For Shrimp Mixture:

3 tablespoons olive oil

1½ pounds medium shrimp, peeled and deveined

12 ounces broccoli florets

8 ounces, carrot, peeled and sliced

Directions:

1. For sauce: in a bowl, place all the ingredients and beat until well combined. Set aside.

2. In a large wok, heat oil over medium-high heat and cook the shrimp for about 2 minutes, stirring occasionally.

3. Add the broccoli and carrot and cook about 3-4 minutes, stirring frequently.

4. Stir in the sauce mixture and cook for about 1-2 minutes.

5. Serve immediately.

Nutrition: Calories 298 Total Fat 10.7 g Saturated Fat 1.3 g Cholesterol 305 mg Sodium 882 mg Total Carbs 7 g Fiber 2g Sugar 2.4 g Protein 45.5 g

23. Chickpeas with Swiss Chard

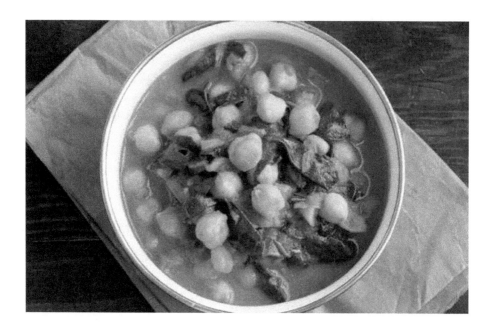

Preparation Time: 15 minutes

Cooking Time: 12 minutes

Servings: 4

Ingredients:

2 tablespoon olive oil

2 garlic cloves, sliced thinly

1 large tomato, chopped finely

2 bunches fresh Swiss chard, trimmed

1 (18-ounce) can chickpeas, drained and rinsed

Salt and ground black pepper, as required

¼ cup of water

1 tablespoon fresh lemon juice

2 tablespoons fresh parsley, chopped

Directions:

1. Heat the oil in a large nonstick wok over medium heat and sauté the garlic for about 1 minute.

2. Add the tomato and cook for about 2-3 minutes, crushing with the back of the spoon.

3. Stir in remaining ingredients except for the lemon juice and parsley and cook for about 5-7 minutes.

4. Drizzle with the lemon juice and remove from the heat.

5. Serve hot with the garnishing of parsley.

Nutrition: Calories 217 Total Fat 8.3 g Saturated Fat 1 g Cholesterol 0 mg Sodium 171 mg Total Carbs 26.2 g Fiber 6.6 g Sugar 1.8 g Protein 8.8 g

24. Buckwheat Noodles with Chicken

Preparation Time: 20 minutes

Cooking Time: 25 minutes

Servings: 2

Ingredients:

½ cup broccoli florets

½ cup fresh green beans, trimmed and sliced

1 cup fresh kale, tough ribs removed and chopped

5 ounces buckwheat noodles

1 tablespoon coconut oil

1 red onion, chopped finely

1 (6-ounce) boneless, skinless chicken breast, cubed

2 garlic cloves, chopped finely

3 tablespoons low-sodium soy sauce

Directions:

1. In a medium pan of the boiling water, add the broccoli and green beans and cook for about 4-5 minutes.

2. Add the kale and cook for about 1-2 minutes.

3. Drain the vegetables and transfer into a large bowl. Set aside.

4. In another pan of the lightly salted boiling water, cook the soba noodles for about 5 minutes.

5. Drain the noodles well and then, rinse under cold running water. Set aside.

6. Meanwhile, in a large wok, melt the coconut oil over medium heat and sauté the onion for about 2-3 minutes.

7. Add the cubes of chicken and cook for approximately 5-6 minutes.

8. Add the garlic, soy sauce and a little splash of water and cook for about 2-3 minutes, stirring frequently.

9. Add the cooked vegetables and noodles and cook for about 1-2 minutes, tossing frequently.

10. Serve hot with the garnishing of sesame seeds.

Nutrition: Calories 463 Total Fat 11.7 g Saturated Fat 5.9 g Cholesterol 54 mg Sodium 1000 mg Total Carbs 58.9 g Fiber 7.1 g Sugar 4.6 g Protein 22.5 g

25. Spicy Sesame & Edamame Noodles

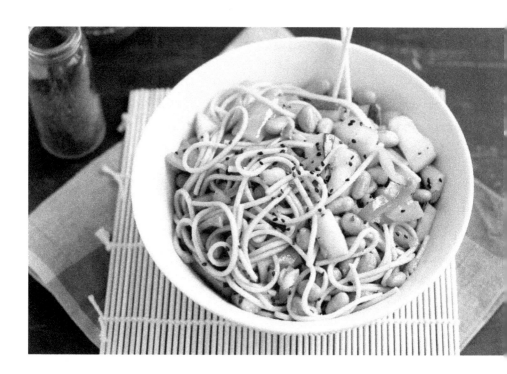

Preparation Time: 5 minutes

Cooking Time: 15 minutes

Servings: 2

Ingredients:

100 g Blue Dragon Whole-wheat Noodles

100 g vegetable 'noodles'

2 tbsp. groundnut or coconut oil

2 shallots, peeled and finely sliced

2 tsp. 'lazy' garlic

2 tsp. ginger puree

1 red chili, sliced

3 tbsp. sesame seeds

100 g edamame beans, podded

2 tbsp. sesame oil

2 tbsp. Blue Dragon soy sauce

Handful fresh coriander, roughly chopped

Juice of 1 lime

Directions:

1. For 4 minutes, boil the noodles, then drain and set aside. Cook the vegetable noodles according to the Directions: and add the rest of the noodles.

2. In a big pan or kettle heat the oil and add garlic, ginger and pepper. Cook for 2 minutes and then add sesame seeds and bean sprouts. Cook for another 2 minutes, stir and stir to make sure nothing sticks to the bottom of the pot.

3. Pour the noodles and the noodles into the pan and cook for 2 minutes.

4. Turn off the heat, then add sesame oil, soy sauce and lemon juice and mix. Serve with scattered coriander.

Nutrition: Calories 230 Carbs 25g Fat 13g Protein 4g

26. Triple Berry Millet Bake

This breakfast bake is full of blueberries, raspberries, and strawberries, which are then complemented with walnuts? Enjoy it alone or with shavings of dark chocolate over the top.

kilocalories Per Individual Serving: 342
The Number of Servings: 8
Time to Prepare/Cook: 70 minutes

The Ingredients:

Millet - 1.5 cups

Soy milk, unsweetened - 2 cups

Water - 1 cup

Date sugar - .5 cup

Vanilla extract - 2 teaspoons

Sea salt - .25 teaspoon

Cinnamon - .5 teaspoon

Walnuts, chopped - 1 cup

Blueberries, thawed if frozen - 12 ounces

Strawberries, sliced, thawed if frozen - 8 ounces

Raspberries, thawed if frozen - 8 ounces

The Directions:

1. Set your oven to Fahrenheit three-hundred and seventy-five degrees and prepare a glass 9-inch by thirteen-inch baking dish.

2. In a large kitchen bowl, whisk together the soy milk, water, millet, date sugar, cinnamon, sea salt, and vanilla extract. Pour the mixture into the prepared pan.

3. Sprinkle the berries and almonds evenly over the top of the pan, and then use a spatula or spoon to slightly press the nuts down into the mixture.

4. Bake the millet until hot and bubbling, about one hour. Remove the millet bake from the oven and allow it to sit for fifteen minutes before serving.

27. Green Shakshuka

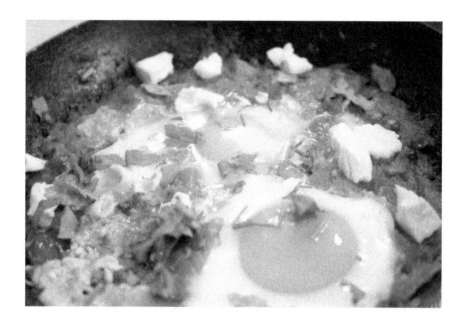

This shakshuka is a twist on the original, with kale, zucchini, Brussels sprouts, and more, to give you a filling and healthy start to your day.

kilocalories Per Individual Serving: 364
The Number of Servings: 3
Time to Prepare/Cook: 17 minutes

The Ingredients:

Zucchini, grated - 1

Brussels sprouts, finely sliced or shaved - 9 ounces

Red onion, diced - 1

Olive oil - 2 tablespoons

Eggs - 5

Parsley, chopped - .25 cup

Kale, chopped - 2 cups

Sea salt - .5 teaspoon

Cumin - 1 teaspoon

Avocado, sliced - 1

The Directions:

1. In large steel, the skillet salutes the red onion in the olive oil until it becomes slightly transparent, about three minutes. Add in the minced garlic and cook the onion/garlic mixture for an additional minute.

2. Add the Brussels sprouts to the skillet containing the onion and garlic, and cook it for four to five minutes until softened, stirring frequently. Stir in the spices and zucchini, cooking for an additional minute.

3. Stir the kale into the skillet and continue to stir until it begins to wilt. Reduce the heat to low.

4. Using a spatula flatten the shakshuka mixture in the skillet and create five small wells for the eggs to next in. Crack an egg

into each of the shakshuka wells and cover the skillet with a lid to steam the eggs until they fit your liking.

5. Top the dish off with the parsley and avocado, serving immediately.

28. Kale and Butternut Bowls

You can easily make the vegetable portion of this dish ahead of time and store it in the fridge or freezer. This will encourage you to reheat it in the mornings easily and serve it with little effort alongside an egg.

kilocalories Per Individual Serving: 324
The Number of Servings: 4
Time to Prepare/Cook: 60 minutes

The Ingredients:
Red onion, diced - 1
Butternut squash, seeds removed and cut into quarters - 1
Kale, chopped - 3 cups
Garlic, minced - 2 cloves
Extra virgin olive oil - 1 tablespoon
Oregano, dried - 1 teaspoon
Cinnamon - .25 teaspoon
Turmeric powder - .5 teaspoon
Sea salt - 1 teaspoon
Avocado, sliced - 1
Eggs - 4
Parsley, chopped - .25 cup
Black pepper, ground - .25 teaspoon

The Directions:

1. Set the oven to Fahrenheit four-hundred and twenty-five degrees. Place the butternut squash on a pan upside-down so that the skin side is facing upward. Roast the butternut squash until it is fork-tender, about twenty-five to thirty minutes.

2. Allow the butternut squash to cool enough to handle easily, and then peel the skin off with your hands. Slice the butternut squash into bite-size cubes.

3. Heat the extra virgin olive oil in a large skillet over medium heat and saute the onion for about five minutes until it is translucent. Add in the kale, garlic, and seasonings, cooking until the kale is wilted. Add in the butternut squash.

4. Divide the skillet mixture between four serving bowls and top each one with an egg cooked to your choice, sliced avocado, and parsley.

29. Egg Casserole

This casserole is full of flavor from your favorite breakfast sausage, vegetables and fresh herbs. You can easily make this at the beginning of the week, and then store it in the fridge for a quick and easy go-to meal.

kilocalories Per Individual Serving: 309
The Number of Servings: 6
Time to Prepare/Cook: 40 minutes

The Ingredients:

Eggs - 10

Breakfast sausage - 1 pound

Button mushrooms, sliced - 2 cups

Roma tomatoes, seeded and diced - 3

Red onion, thinly sliced - 1

Kale, chopped - 2 cups

Basil, chopped - 1 tablespoon

Parsley, chopped - 2 tablespoons

Sea salt - 1.5 teaspoons

The Directions:

1. Set your oven to Fahrenheit three-hundred and fifty degrees and prepare a nine-inch by thirteen-inch baking dish.

2. In a skillet over medium-high brown, your breakfast sausage until fully cooked, draining off any excess fat.

3. Into the skillet with the breakfast sausage, add the mushrooms, allowing them to saute until tender, about five to seven minutes. Add in the sea salt and remaining vegetables, cooking for an additional two to three minutes until just slightly tender.

4. Transfer the vegetable sausage mixture to the prepared pan.

5. Whisk together the eggs in a large bowl, ensuring the whites fully break down into the yolks. Pour the eggs over the breakfast sausage and mix vegetables, then placing it in the oven to roast until cooked through, about twenty-five to thirty minutes.

30. Vegan Tofu Omelet

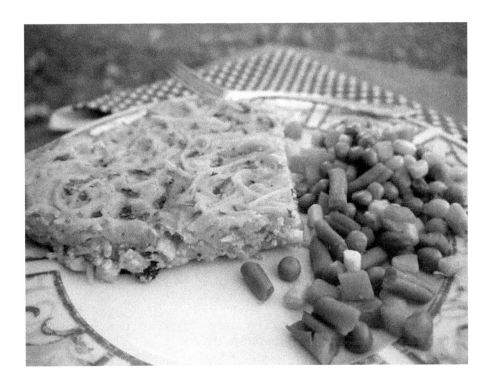

This vegan omelet uses tofu to create an egg-like texture, and black salt to give it an egg-like flavor. You can buy black salt online and at specialty stores. If you can't find black salt, you can replace it with regular sea salt, but know it won't have the same egg-like flavor.

kilocalories Per Individual Serving: 276
The Number of Servings: 1
Time to Prepare/Cook: 15 minutes

The Ingredients:

Silken tofu - 6 ounces Tahini - 1 teaspoon (optional)

Cornstarch - 1 tablespoon

Nutritional yeast - 1 tablespoon

Soy milk, unsweetened - 1 tablespoon

Turmeric, ground - .125 teaspoon

Onion powder - .25 teaspoon

Sea salt - .25 teaspoon

Smoked paprika - .125 teaspoon (optional)

Black salt - .25 teaspoon

Kale, chopped - .5 cup

Button mushrooms, sliced - .25 cup

Onion, diced - 2 tablespoons

Garlic, minced - 1 clove

Extra virgin olive oil - 1 tablespoon, dived

The Directions:

1. Into a blender, add the tofu, tahini, cornstarch, yeast, soy milk, turmeric, onion powder, smoked paprika, and bath salts.Pulse on high until fully blended with the mixture.

2. In a skillet, add half of the olive oil along with the vegetables and garlic. Saute until they become tender, about five minutes over medium heat.

3. Meanwhile, add the remaining half of the olive oil to a non-stick medium skillet over medium-high heat. Allow this skillet to preheat while you cook the vegetables until it is very hot. Once hot, pour the tofu batter into the skillet, slightly tilting the pan so that the egg forms a circular shape. You can use a spoon to smooth out the top.

4. Sprinkle the cooked vegetables over the tofu "egg" and reduce the heat of the skillet to medium-low. Cover the skillet with a lid, allowing it to cook three to five minutes until the tofu "egg" is set and the edges have dried. You can use a spatula to lightly lift the edges of the omelet and ensure it is fully set. The coloring should be golden with some browned spots.

5. When ready, loosen the omelet by lifting it with the spatula and then flip one side over the other. Transfer the tofu omelet to a plate and enjoy while warm.

31. Grapefruit & Celery Blast

Ingredients

1 grapefruit, peeled

2 stalks of celery

50g (2oz) kale

½ teaspoon matcha powder

71 calories per serving

The Number of Servings: 1

The Directions:

1. Place all the ingredients into a blender with enough water to cover them and blitz until smooth.

32. Orange & Celery Crush

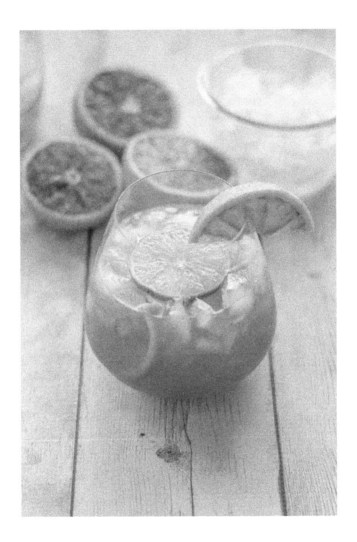

Ingredients

1 carrot, peeled

3 stalks of celery

1 orange, peeled

½ teaspoon matcha powder

Juice of 1 lime

95 calories per serving

The Number of Servings: 1

The Directions:

1. Place all of the ingredients into a blender with enough water to cover them and blitz until smooth.

33. Tropical Chocolate Delight

Ingredients

1 mango, peeled & de-stoned

75g (3oz) fresh pineapple, chopped

50g (2oz) kale

25g (1oz) rocket

1 tablespoon 100% cocoa powder or cacao nibs 150mls (5fl oz) coconut milk

427 calories per serving

The Number of Servings: 1

The Directions:

1. Place all of the ingredients into a blender and blitz until smooth. When it seems too thick, you should add a little water.

34. Walnut & Spiced Apple Tonic

Ingredients

6 walnuts halves

1 apple, cored

1 banana

½ teaspoon matcha powder

½ teaspoon cinnamon

Pinch of ground nutmeg

272 calories per serving

The Number of Servings: 1

The Directions:

1. Place all of the ingredients into a blender and add sufficient water to cover them. Blitz until smooth and creamy.

35. Sweet Rocket (Arugula) Boost

Ingredients

25g (1oz) fresh rocket (arugula) leaves

75g (3oz) kale

1 apple

1 carrot

1 tablespoon fresh parsley

Juice of 1 lime

113 calories per serving

The Number of Servings: 1

The Directions:

1.   Place all of the ingredients into a blender with enough water to cover and process until smooth.

36. Banana & Ginger Snap

Ingredients

2.5cm (1 inch) chunk of fresh ginger, peeled

1 banana

1 large carrot

1 apple, cored

½ stick of celery

¼ level teaspoon turmeric powder

166 calories per serving

The Number of Servings: 1

The Directions:

1. Place all the ingredients into a blender with just enough water to cover them.

2. Process until smooth

37. Chocolate, Strawberry & Coconut Crush

Ingredients

100mls (3½fl oz) coconut milk

100g (3½oz) strawberries

1 banana

1 tablespoon 100% cocoa powder or cacao nibs

1 teaspoon matcha powder

324 calories per serving

The Number of Servings: 1

The Directions:

1. Toss all of the ingredients into a blender and process them to a creamy consistency. Add a little additional water if you need to thin it out a little.

38. Chocolate Berry Blend

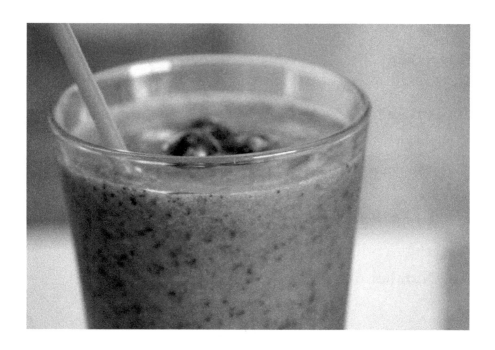

Ingredients

50g (2oz) kale

50g (2oz) blueberries

50g (2oz) strawberries

1 banana

1 tablespoon 100% cocoa powder or cacao nibs 200mls (7fl oz) unsweetened soya milk

241 calories per serving

The Number of Servings: 1

The Directions:

1.   Place all of the ingredients into a blender with enough water to cover them and process until smooth.

39. Cranberry & Kale Crush

Ingredients

75g (3oz) strawberries

 50g (2oz) kale

120mls (4fl oz) unsweetened cranberry juice 1 teaspoon chia seeds

½ teaspoon matcha powder

71 calories per serving

The Number of Servings: 1

The Directions:

1. Place all of the ingredients into a blender and process until smooth. Add some crushed ice and a mint leaf or two for a refreshing drink.

40. Poached Eggs & Rocket (Arugula)

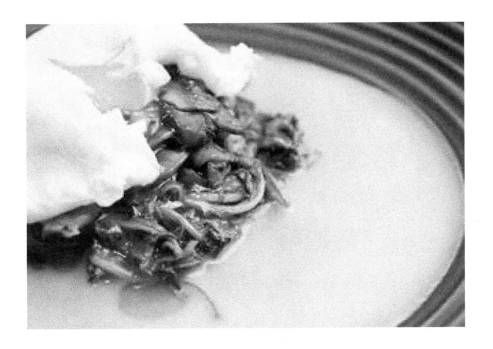

Ingredients

2 eggs

25g (1oz) fresh rocket (arugula)

1 teaspoon olive oil

Sea salt

Freshly ground black pepper 178 calories per serving

The Number of Servings: 1

The Directions:

1. Scatter the rocket (arugula) leaves onto a plate and drizzle the olive oil over them. Bring a shallow pan of water to the boil, Put the eggs in and cook until the whites are strong. Serve the eggs on top of the rocket and season with salt and pepper.

41. Strawberry Buckwheat Pancakes

Ingredients

100g (3½oz) strawberries, chopped

100g (3½ oz) buckwheat flour

1 egg

250mls (8fl oz) milk

1 teaspoon olive oil

1 teaspoon olive oil for frying

Freshly squeezed juice of 1 orange

175 calories per serving

The Number of Servings: 4

The Directions:

1. Pour the milk into a bowl and mix in the egg and a teaspoon of olive oil. Sift in the flour to the liquid mixture until smooth and creamy. Allow it to rest for 15 minutes. Heat a little oil in a pan and pour in a quarter of the mixture (or to the size you prefer.) Sprinkle in a quarter of the strawberries into the batter—Cook for around 2 minutes on each side. Serve hot with a drizzle of orange juice. You could try experimenting with other berries such as blueberries and blackberries.

42. Strawberry & Nut Granola

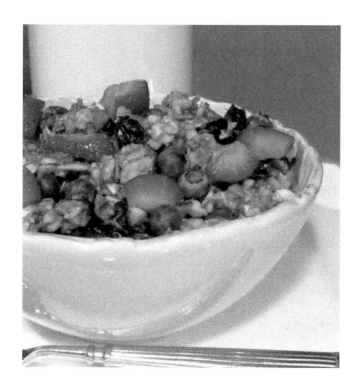

Ingredients

200g (7oz) oats

250g (9oz) buckwheat flakes

100g (3½ oz) walnuts, chopped

100g (3½ oz) almonds, chopped

100g (3½ oz) dried strawberries

1½ teaspoons ground ginger

1½ teaspoons ground cinnamon

120mls (4fl oz) olive oil

2 tablespoon honey

391 calories per serving

The Number of Servings: 12

The Directions:

1. Combine the oats, buckwheat flakes, nuts, ginger and cinnamon. In a saucepan, warm the oil and honey,. Stir until the honey has melted. Pour the warm oil into the dry ingredients and mix well. Spread the mixture out on a large baking tray (or two) and bake in the oven at 150C (300F) for around 50 minutes until the granola is golden. Allow it to cool. Add in the dried berries. Store in an airtight container until ready to use. Can be served with yogurt, milk or even dry as a handy snack.

43. Chilled Strawberry & Walnut Porridge

Ingredients

100g (3½ oz) strawberries

50g (2oz) rolled oats

4 walnut halves, chopped

1 teaspoon chia seeds

200mls (7fl oz) unsweetened soya milk 100ml (3½ fl oz) water

384 calories

The Number of Servings: 1

The Directions:

1. Place the strawberries, oats, soya milk and water into a blender and process until smooth. Stir in the chia seeds and mix well. Chill in the fridge overnight and serve in the morning with a sprinkling of chopped walnuts. It's simple and delicious.

44. Fruit & Nut Yogurt Crunch

Ingredients

100g (3½ oz) plain Greek yogurt

50g (2oz) strawberries, chopped

6 walnut halves, chopped

The sprinkling of cocoa powder

296 calories

The Number of Servings: 1

The Directions:

1. Stir half of the chopped strawberries into the yogurt. Using a glass, place a layer of yogurt with a sprinkling of strawberries and walnuts, followed by another layer of the same until you reach the top of the glass.

2. Garnish with walnuts pieces and a dusting of cocoa powder.

45. Cheesy Baked Eggs

Ingredients

4 large eggs

75g (3oz) cheese, grated

25g (1oz) fresh rocket (arugula) leaves, finely chopped

1 tablespoon parsley

½ teaspoon ground turmeric

1 tablespoon olive oil

198 calories per serving

The Number of Servings: 4

The Directions:

1. Grease each ramekin dish with a little olive oil. Divide the rocket (arugula) between the ramekin dishes then break an egg into each one. Sprinkle a little parsley and turmeric on top then sprinkle on the cheese. In a preheated oven, place the ramekins at220C/425F for 15 minutes, until the eggs are set and the cheese is bubbling.

46. Spiced Scramble

Ingredients

25g (1oz) kale, finely chopped

2 eggs

1 spring onion (scallion) finely chopped

1 teaspoon turmeric

1 tablespoon olive oil

Sea salt

Freshly ground black pepper 259 calories per serving

The Number of Servings: 1

The Directions:

1. Crack the eggs into a bowl. Add the turmeric and whisk them— season with salt and pepper. Heat the oil in a frying pan, add the kale and spring onions (scallions) and cook until it has wilted. Pour in the beaten eggs and stir until eggs have scrambled together with the kale.

47. Sirtfood Mushroom Scramble Eggs

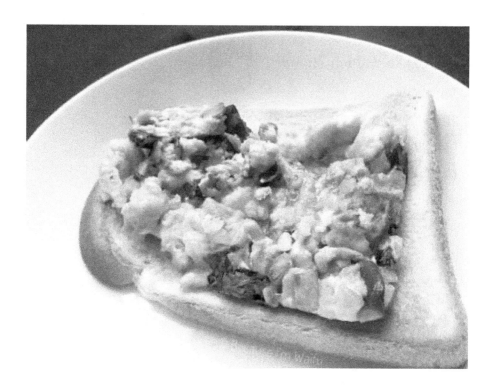

Ingredients

2 tbsp.

1 teaspoon ground garlic

1 teaspoon mild curry powder

20g lettuce, approximately sliced

1 teaspoon extra virgin olive oil

1/2 bird's eye peeled, thinly chopped

A couple of mushrooms, finely chopped 5g parsley, finely chopped *elective * insert a seed mix for a topper plus some rooster sauce for taste

The Directions:

1. Mix the curry and garlic powder and then add just a little water till you've achieved a light glue.

2. Steam the lettuce for two -- 3 minutes.

3. Eat the oil over a moderate heat in a skillet and fry the chili and mushrooms 2-3 minutes till they've begun to soften and brown.

4. Insert the eggs and spice paste and cook over moderate heat, then add the carrot and then proceed to cook over a moderate heat for a further minute. In the end, put in the parsley, mix well, and function.

48. Blue Hawaii Smoothie

Ingredients

2 tablespoons ring or approximately 4-5 balls 1/2 cup frozen tomatoes

Two tbsp ground flaxseed

⅛ cup tender coconut (unsweetened, organic)

Few walnuts

1/2 cup fat-free yogurt

5-6 ice cubes Dab of water

The Directions:

1. Throw all of the ingredients together and combine until smooth. You might need to prevent and wake up to receive it combined smoothie or put in more water.

49. Turkey Breakfast Sausages

Ingredients

1 lb. extra lean ground turkey

1 tbsp. EVOO, and a little more to dirt pan

1 tbsp. fennel seeds

1 teaspoon smoked paprika

1 teaspoon red pepper flakes

1 teaspoon peppermint

1 teaspoon chicken seasoning

A couple of shredded cheddar cheese

A couple of chives, finely chopped

A few shakes garlic and onion powder

Two spins of pepper and salt

The Directions:

1. Preheat oven to 350f.

2. Utilize a little EVOO to dirt a miniature muffin pan.

3. Combine all ingredients and blend thoroughly.

4. Fill each pit on top of the pan and then cook for approximately 15-20 minutes. Each toaster differs; therefore, when muffin fever is 165, then remove.

50. Banana Pecan Muffins

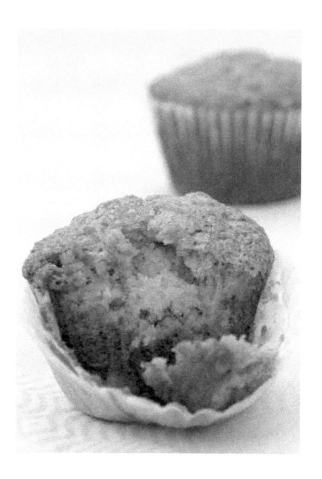

Ingredients

3 tbsp. butter softened

3 ripe bananas

1 tbsp. honey

⅛ cup oj

1 teaspoon cinnamon

1 cups all-purpose pasta

2 capsules

A couple of pecans, sliced

1 tbsp. vanilla

The Directions:

1. Preheat the oven to 180°c/ / 350°f.

2. Lightly grease the muffin tin's bottom and sides, and then dust with flour.

3. Dust the surfaces of the tin gently with flour then tap to eradicate any excess.

4. Peel and insert the batter to a mixing bowl and with a fork, mash the carrots; therefore that you've got a combination of chunky and smooth, then put aside.

5. Insert the orange juice, melted butter, eggs, vanilla, and spices and stir to combine.

6. Roughly chop the pecans onto a chopping board, when using, then fold throughout the mix.

7. Spoon at the batter 3/4 full and bake in the oven for approximately 40 minutes, or until golden and cooked through.

CPSIA information can be obtained
at www.ICGtesting.com
Printed in the USA
BVHW041010150321
602551BV00006B/369